I0791766

Sheena C. Pickett

PRESENTS

Raw Footage

A Gentlemen's Guide to Proper Foot Care

Raw Footage: A Gentlemen's Guide to Proper Foot Care

Sheena Pickett

Printed in the United States of America

We gratefully acknowledge the editing contribution of Monique S. Shields and Legacy Publishing LLC.

This book or parts thereof may not be reproduced in any form, stored in a retrieval system, or transmitted in any form by any means —electronic, mechanical, photocopy, recording, or otherwise —without the expressed written consent of the publisher, except as provided by United States of America copyright law.

Copyright © 2017 by Sheena C. Pickett
All rights reserved

Book Outline

Shout Outs

To my Parents,

Mother, Rickie and Pops

I Love You

To my Triangle Offense,

Sterling Green

You are my strength when it is low

LeMond Crayton-Hart

I pinky promised

Monique Shields

My life would be "the blob" without you

Table of Contents

THE STARTING LINEUP

"How you describe your FEET is a direct reflection of the LIFE you live!"- Sheena Pickett

I've been inspired by the facets of holistic care for over a decade, but the vision of "Raw Footage: A Gentlemen's Guide to Proper Foot Care." is something that I've carried for longer than I can remember. The Universe has a way of putting me at the right place, surrounded by the right people at the right time. During meditation, I occasionally replay my life -like a good book that needs to be reread. Knowing that there was something I must have missed the first time. Taking notes, underlining, and highlighting possible clues to how I got here. Going from chapter to chapter, paragraph to paragraph, sentence to sentence, from words to letters. My life, this book, my business and love of service would not have been possible without yielding to each clue.

Each clue was another step and each one of my steps are and have been strategically ordered to bring me to a place of understanding. I am grateful to accept my purpose. But don't get it twisted...there are levels to this staircase with a few broken, squeaky and missing steps along the way. The hardest levels I've had to master were trusting the process and the ability to be patient beyond worry. Oftentimes Fear and worrying often block solutions and hold your time hostage. The key to unlocking the lessons came in the form of relationships. One major key was understanding that relationships are a direct reflection of me.

Relationships are important, especially between men and women. My first relationship with an AlphaMale was with my Pops. My Father is a provider, giver of wisdom, the epitome of strength, a hustler and a leader. The father-daughter relationship is vital for every woman. That relationship allowed me to be comfortable in my humility. Feeling protected in that capacity empowering me to own my commitment to service and my gift as a practitioner.

Today my gift has certainly put me before great men and I am truly grateful. As I grow through this journey of life, my perspective of men consistently evolves. I can honestly say I've had the opportunity to engage with a diverse group of men daily for quite some time; and I'm not talking about just simple chit-chat or 180 characters or less. I'm talking real, meaningful, conversations about wives, exes, drama, side-chicks and children, their dreams and disappointments, wins and losses that turn into lessons.

It's a privilege to listen and learn life from an often-distant perspective. These perspectives add tremendous value, but are often under-appreciated or at best, misunderstood.

Men are a powerful force needed in our lives, communities, and families. Somewhere between co-parenting and career goals, the priority of self-care for most men has been totally dismissed. In efforts to uplift our fallen heroes, I chose to launch a series of products and services that encourage them to stand strong and embrace the path.

RAW FOOTAGE is designed to educate readers and foster a greater appreciation for feet and their purpose. In this book, you will find practical ways for preserving the foundation upon which we all stand. Your feet have been with you since day one. They are your clues. They know where you've been, where you are and where you're headed. Putting your best foot forward encompasses every aspect of your lives: financially, spiritually, physically, and emotionally!

This book helps us explore the anatomy and structure of the feet as I cover popular ailments shared amongst men and strategies on how to alleviate them. Together we'll take an exclusive peak into the importance of essential oils and how you can create practical blends and recipes that are complementary to your grooming regiment. We'll discover how our feet relate to many principles that govern our faith. Then we're headed deep into the *man cave* to eradicate fear and help travelers detail their approach to life and redefine their masculinity.

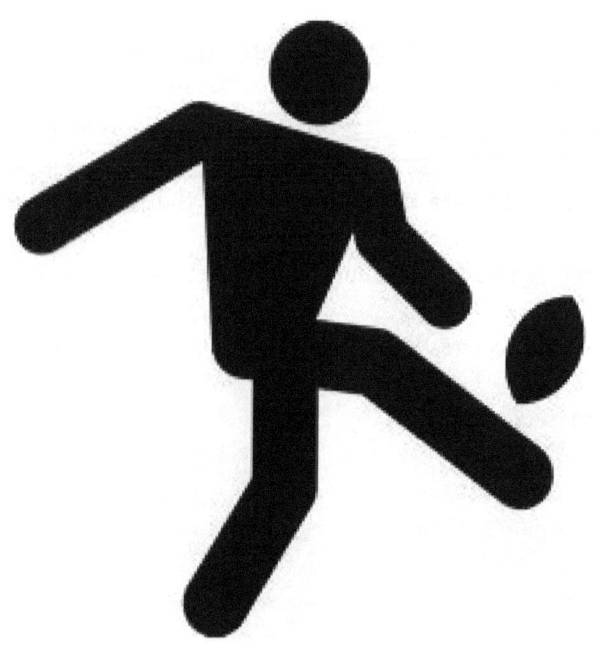

KICKOFF

Client (Feet)back and Review

"So let me tell y'all about my first time and how it finally went down. I know from what you all know or assume, you think that it may go down for me all the time but that's not the case. It had to be the right time and with someone I was comfortable with. Anyways when I came into her space, I let her know this was new to me, she said ok just relax, take off some clothing and let her handle it. I said ok but she sensed my nervousness so she caressed my hand and served me up. Since it was our first encounter there was a rough start but we soon settled into a rhythmic groove. I reclined back and man she was amazing!!! Made my toes curl good. I had no ego in complimenting her skills and talents, the hand job was out of this world. She handled my size and girth like a champ. Basically, from my fingertips to the edge my toes, the sister handled business...which is why I am urging all my fellas for your manicure and pedicure needs...holla at AlphaMale Nail Care Services and my girl Sheena!!!"

Submitted December 31, 2016

@Patrickeward via Facebook

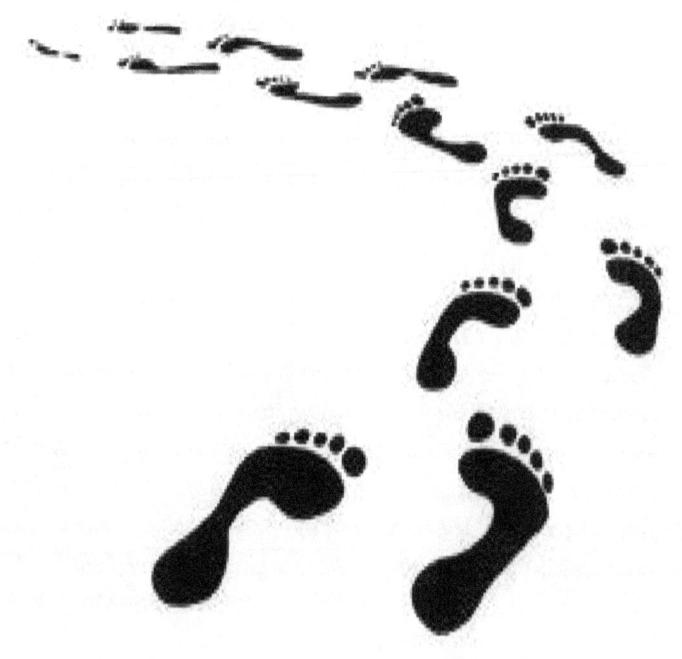

FOOT TRAFFIC

*"The journey of thousand miles begins
with a single step." -Lao Tzu*

Every structure in history, every invention, idea, object, etc....has a foundation. For us, I'd like to think our foundation begins with our FEET!! Imagine a life without the use of our feet. Of course, modern advances in technology and prosthetics have provided solutions to such dilemmas; but just reflect for a second on all the morning activities that take place before we leave our homes to start our day. Waking up, getting out of bed, walking to the bathroom, showering, dressing, going to the kitchen to make breakfast and driving off to work. I know that is a very brief excerpt of typical morning mayhem, but imagine filling in the blanks with your typical morning activities and doing it without the use of your feet.

I often tell my clients "take care of your feet because you only get one set". More often than not, my more mature aka elderly clients mention that they wish they had taken better care of their feet. As we age, we tend to neglect the tools that have carried us through our journey called Life. With all that we've got going on foot care is the least of our priorities. And we never quite take the time to appreciate them as we should. I completely get it!! Our first impressions don't include our feet, but what gets the most play is what's on our feet, the wardrobe, haircut, and physique.

It's said that the average moderately active person takes around 7500 steps per day, I can verify that with this Fitbit. Maintaining that daily average and an average lifespan of 80 years you'll have walked about 216,262,500 steps in your lifetime. Those that know me know that I'm about the numbers so-much-so that I dedicated 4.5 years of my life to receiving a

B.A in mathematics...so you can guarantee the math is accurate. Having said that, the average person would have walked about 110,000 miles, which is the equivalent of walking about 5x around the Earth's equator. That's a lot of foot traffic...no pun intended. But you get the point, our feet are powerful machines of movement and a vital part of our existence. Aiding and carrying us along our voyage of experiences. "Raw Footage: The Gentlemen's Guide to Proper Foot Care" is just a road-map to help give instruction for a more pleasant passage.

FOOT FETISH

*"The Human Foot is a Masterpiece of engineering
and a work of art." -Leonardo da Vinci*

Just go with me on this...think of your feet as the body of a beautiful woman from head to toe. Her movement, flexibility, and mechanics are all quite sexy and engaging especially if you take the time and study it. Now that I've gotten your attention...let's keep it going. The curves, lines, and symmetry have a design like no other. It may sound like I have sort of a foot fetish and that *may* be true, but over time I've just gained a great appreciation for feet. And I totally believe it's much better to think about feet in this manner than in terms of bunions, cracked heels or corns and callus' (we'll get to that later). If you think of your feet as a beautiful curvaceous work of art, similar to your vehicle, you'll learn to respect them a little more. Or from the famous Birdman interview, you'll "put some *respeck* on it" and hopefully begin to treat them better.

There are 26 bones in the foot, divided into 3 sections. Those three sections are the forefoot, midfoot, and hindfoot. The forefoot is like the face of that attractive woman we spoke of earlier with piercing eyes, a soft slender nose, full voluptuous lips, a smooth and sexy chin with an elongated neck that trails down to round firm breast. The midfoot is the alluring abdomen with a narrow waist and section three the hindfoot is the mesmerizing hips that don't lie. The 26 bones of both feet make up about one-fourth of the 206 bones in the body. These bones work with 31 joints, connected by 107 ligaments and 36 muscles. To sum it up, our feet are kind-of a big deal. They absorb the shock of walking or running; Bending and flexing as they carry and support the weight of our bodies from destination to destination. Our feet are incredible and

wonderfully made!

INJURY REPORT: (GUY)DELINES

"Injuries are part of the game, but sometimes we can avoid them by just practicing our techniques."
-Troy Vincent

Not a day passes that doesn't include my favorite ESPN show "First Take" with Stephen A. Smith and Skip Bayless who was recently replaced by Max Kellerman. As the commentators share their opinions and debate the latest headlines about players, coaches, and drama both on and off the field; it never fails that injuries are always a part of the conversation. How many times have you heard of an athlete being out for the season or several weeks due to stress fractures, plantar fasciitis, ankle sprain, torn Achilles or something fractured, twisted, irritated, or ruptured? These injuries will fuck up your fantasy football rankings and have your favorite player contemplating retirement.

During sports or other strenuous activities and workouts, the pressure applied to the body, more specifically the feet, can reach up to 10 times your body weight. Overuse and the lack of proper stretching result in men being more susceptible to foot injuries. Let's discuss a few of these injuries in depth:

Plantar Fasciitis

What do Albert Pujols, Antonio Gates, Peyton Manning, Pau Gasol and Joakim Noah, all have in common – besides being recognized as superior athletes in their respective sport? These players have suffered in one way or another from plantar fasciitis.

Literary knocking athletes off their feet, plantar fasciitis is micro tears in the band of tissues that connect the heel bone to the toe. Over time these tears develop throughout the tissue along the bottom of the foot causing it to become inflamed, swollen and tender. Usually, pain is felt within the first few steps out the bed in the morning along with a burst of pain throughout the day. Plantar Fasciitis usually develops in an active individual that participate in quick sudden movements that are overly repetitive, such as the movements demonstrated in playing basketball and running or sprinting.

A few at home remedies to prevent and possibly reverse plantar fasciitis include: calf and toe stretching and pulling your toes towards you with your hands until you feel the stretch of the ball of your foot. One of my favorite techniques to perform for my clients during the "Athlete's Pedicure" is making use of a small ball, a golf or a tennis ball will do. I begin by rolling the golf ball along the bottom of the feet gently to massage and loosen up the plantar fascia. Next, continue by taking the ball and roll it up and down the lower calf and around the ankle to help alleviate muscle tension. The next technique I call "Ice Up Son" which utilizes ice to help with controlling the inflammation. Taking the same action mentioned earlier with a small ball you can repurpose a water bottle that's been frozen and effectively keep things loose and the swelling in check.

Maintaining consistency with these tips and techniques over the course of a few weeks will help to alleviate the pain and reduce inflammation.

Heel Spurs

Heel spurs are a byproduct of plantar fasciitis as well. They are deposits of calcium that lodges itself on the heel due to tension and inflammation from plantar fascia (bands of tissue). It does not produce any pain but is the visible evidence that shows up on the x-ray to indicate that the patient has plantar fasciitis. Heel spurs outwardly produce bony overgrowths on the heel bone. Heel spurs develop due to inadequate flexibility, being overweight or having high arches.

Solutions to treat heel spurs are to remove the pressure by lodging padding or cushions inside the shoes. Although painful, massaging the area of discomfort has proven to be successful when done daily for a couple of weeks.

Bunions

Bunions are like "Hump Day" on the big toe. It's when a bony hump grows on the joint of the toe. Various causes are ill-fitted and narrow shoes, genetics, poor running habits that are influenced by over/under pronation, or the misalignment of the big toe. Because bunions rest on the joint where the toe bends, bunions can be extremely painful with each step. To alleviate the pain, wear roomy shoes that have wide and deep toe boxes and have good arch support. Avoid or adjust activities that apply pressure to the big toe or foot. If these nonsurgical treatments don't relieve your pain, surgery can be the last resort that corrects the deformed area near the big toe.

Achilles Tendonitis

Sports Illustrated reported that 70% of all Achilles Tendon ruptures occur during sports with quick repetitive movement like those within basketball, soccer, tennis or running. Most of these injuries occur within middle-aged, male weekend warriors, during the spring and summer months. You know… the ones holding on to their hoop dreams from high school. Reminiscing about the buzzer beater shot that could have changed his life had it not been for a bad referee call. Or those that sporadically work out but tend to do too much, too quick, too soon during a Saturday pickup game.

Achilles is an injury to the Achilles tendon, which connects the calf muscle to the heel bone. Tendonitis occurs when excessive force and intensity over a period-of-time strains the calf muscle and becomes painfully inflamed. You'll know somethings up if there is swelling in the back of your heel, calf muscles feel tight and limited ROM (range of motion) when flexing the foot. Also the skin on the heel feels overly warm to the touch. But some good news is that most cases can be remedied with a little

R.I.C.E: Rest, Ice, Compression, and Elevation

R – Rest

Rest and reduce your physical activity. Don't apply pressure or weight on the tendon for a couple of days. The tendon will usually heal faster with no additional strain being placed on it during this time.

I – Icing

Ice the area after exercise or when in pain. Ice will usually make the inflammation or swelling decrease within a 15 or 20-minute time frame.

C- Compress

Compress the injury with a bandage or an article of clothing. Compression will keep the tendon from continuously swelling. Try not to tie or wrap too tight as this will limit blood flow.

E – Elevate

Elevate your foot above the level of your chest. When your foot is higher than your heart the blood flows back to the heart and thus keeps the swelling down. But if the tendon has ruptured or torn you have no choice except to see a doctor for surgery.

Some methods to reduce and prevent the risk of injury:

- Stretch your calf muscles often to improve agility and strength especially before and after workouts.

- Be easy when it comes to new exercise routines and intensify your physical activity gradually.

- Mix it up and cross train...combine high and low impact exercises to work a variety of muscles and alleviate stress and overuse of the same tendons.

- Choose shoes with proper cushioning and arch support and rotate between different pairs of shoes throughout the week.

Second Strings

I don't like to be repetitive or maybe I'm just being lazy but throughout this chapter, I'll drop some "Second Strings". These are ailments that are similar in remedy and cause as those mentioned in full detail.

Second String: Stress Fractures (See Achilles Tendonitis)

Stress Fractures are tiny cracks in the bone caused by repetitive stress or force, often from overuse or from activities that require lots of running and jumping.

Callous, Corns and Cracked Heels

We are all familiar with Callus. It's the thick and ugly tough area of skin that forms due to repeated friction and pressure. Most commonly found on feet and hands; Callus is like your skins cape of protection from ill-fitted shoes or arm day at the gym. I tell my clients all the time callus is the gift that keeps on giving. Hear me out...cutting callus is the worst thing to do, it's arrogant and will come back stronger and tougher. Instead of cutting you should smooth callus with a pumice stone or emery board. If you have no clue what a pumice stone is google it or ask the nearest woman present. Afterwards, moisturize the area to keep it soft and manageable. The best time is right after showering. If you don't have good moisturizers and want to stop borrowing your girl's stuff...keep reading I will share household recipes to help keep feet and hands at their best. These various ointments help heal various foot ailments and conditions, designed JUST FOR MEN and are all natural.

If you take nothing else from this section remember that no one likes being caressed or touched with rough, dry, sandpaper-like hands. Whether in a handshake or lying in bed with your lady; It's unattractive and can be a hindrance to further training. I would highly recommend wearing gloves during arm and back day but I know that's not going to happen. But as an alternative consider wearing leather hand grips, chalk it up and regularly treat yourself to a monthly manicure. But the key is to be consistent with whichever method you choose.

Second String: Corns (See Callus)

Corns are tiny circular callus that develops between toes. Most commonly associated with ill-fitted foot wear, wearing shoes without socks, and standing for a long period of time in those shoes. I know fashion and a well-coordinated outfit is a big deal but you've got to protect your foundation and when you do it will take care of you!

Second String: Cracked Heels (See Callus)

Cracked heels are a common foot problem. Caused by dry callus skin that is so thick and lacking moisture it begins to crack like dry mud in the desert. Think of pressing your hand on top of a fully ripe tomato sitting on a kitchen counter. As it expands outwardly under the pressure of your hand, the skin begins to split. This similar effect takes place on the fatty pad of flesh on the bottom of the heel due to prolonged standing and being overweight. Suitable solutions in addition to those mentioned in treating callus are to

- avoid open heel shoes

- seek the help of a podiatrist to understand the source of the problem and have them prescribe a medicated ointment

- use insoles to help alter your walking patterns or a heel cup that helps to contain the "fat pad" from splitting.

Athlete's Foot

What do mushrooms and athletes foot have in common? Imagine your foot is a tree in the middle of a dark, wet and warm rainforest. This rainforest is your shoes and your toes are the roots of this tree. Mushrooms, also known as fungi usually grow near the roots of wet trees. When fungus is growing on your feet it makes its home between your toes. The skin on the foot reacts to this growth with itching and redness, cracking and odor. This is Athlete's foot also known as "foot mushrooms", you'll never look at Portobello's the same.

Athlete's foot is a contagious fungal skin infection that flourishes in locker rooms, shower floors, poolside or just having wet feet that are exposed to the fungus. Athletes foot is curable but annoying. If not properly treated it can spread and lead to bacterial infection. Some preventative measures, when exposed to potential threats of athlete's foot, are to wear shower shoes. The cracks and crevices of these public facilities are a perfect habitat for fungus. And if your skin is cracked along the foot you'll be unable to protect yourself. Public showers are the number one location to find athlete's foot fungus. After spending time in these locations clean your shower shoes with apple cider vinegar or baking soda. As stated earlier these products help eliminate bacteria and fungus. Also upon returning home, allow shower shoes, Nike slides or flip-flops to air out on the patio. Wash your feet thoroughly with a scrubbing action because shower shoes are fitted; feet can become sweaty while confined within these shoes. Afterwards, pay close attention to drying the surface of your feet and in between toes. Please be mindful to immediately wash and clean towels and wash your hand to discontinue the spread of the fungus to other materials and other areas of the body.

In general, shoes should be routinely aired out and you should switch between different pairs of shoes throughout the week to allow one pair a break for 24 hours. Baking soda can be used as a foot soak as well as sprinkled within shoes to freshen up stinky shoes and absorb moisture. Another vital measure to protect yourself against athlete's foot is to keep toenails short and clean. Nails that extend past the toe can house and spread infection. If athlete's foot has spread uncontrollably it's time to see a doctor. Treatments prescribed could be OTC that can be taken topically or orally. These treatments generally take 2 -6 weeks for symptoms to disappear.

Men have a higher chance of getting athlete's foot 2 to 4 times as much as women. But it's simple to decrease your risk of exposure. Cleaning with chlorine bleach and household cleaners that kill mold help tremendously.

Discoloration & Thickening Toenails

Every two weeks I make a visit to senior living communities and provide mobile in-house nail care services to the residents. The wisdom and conversation I'm exposed to during these services are priceless. Shared wisdom from personal anecdotes learned from years of living, expressed joy about graduating grandchildren to juicy intel concerning the in-laws and neighboring residents. It's never a dull moment!! But the one commonality with these aging clients is they wish they would have taken better care of their feet. I completely understand...your feet are the last thing on the to-do list when it comes to life, children, and career. As time passes we don't realize that throughout our journey are feet have traveled the distance along with us.

As a manicurist that caters to the elderly, I noticed that thick and discolored toenails were a problem that most residents wanted a solution for. Naturally, as we age toenail discoloration and thickening take place. But disease, trauma, and fungus play a major role as well. Let's explore these causes more in-depth.

Trauma/Injury

Trauma can be described as dropping a couch on your foot while trying to help a homie move into his new place or simply the repetitive pressure of walking and striking your toenail against the top of your shoes. Generally, any alteration to the actual nail or the nail bed (the flesh that the nail lays upon) technically called the matrix; can cause the nail to become thick. This thickness happens because of poor circulation: nerve ending and/or cells in this area have been damaged and lack nourishment. Once damage has occurred to the matrix the nail attached will not go back to normal.

Fungus

Do you recall the portobello aka foot mushrooms? Fungal infection is a major cause of thickening toenails and is visible on the nail by changing in texture and color from a fleshy pink pigment to green, brown, and/or yellow. Also, separation of the nail from the toe, foul odor and the development of fluid are signs of fungus. Stated earlier in describing athlete's foot; fungus thrives in warm, dark and damp environments.

You can develop a fungal nail infection in a variety of ways. Some such cases are those that have diabetes, those who enjoy public swimming pools and locker rooms, and those failing to thoroughly dry hands and feet after washing them and wearing tight closed- toe shoes.

Disease

Disease such as psoriasis, eczema, rheumatoid arthritis, diabetes, cardiovascular disease, etc. may affect toenails. These ailments restrict the flow of blood that circulates throughout the body and to the lower extremities. Also, the medication associated with treating these illnesses can have side effects that weaken the immune system. Similar to hair, nail abnormalities usually stem from malnutrition and vitamin deficiency.

Because hair and nails are made of the same protein called keratin; medication tends to alter nutrient levels and therefore change the appearance, color, shape, texture, and thickness of nails. The health of your nails can be a clue to detect disease through its color. Nail discoloration can be an early diagnosis of lung, heart, kidney, and liver diseases as well as diabetes and anemia.

Ingrown Toenails

One of the frequent questions my clients ask me often is: What is the worst thing I've dealt with concerning men's feet? At this point, I haven't seen anything that has caused me to update my resume and get back to the corporate ladder. But there was an incident when a guest had not cut his toenails in over a year and they began to cuff his toe like a fitted cap. Check out the background story on how he ended up in front of me for a pedicure! It started 2 years earlier...from a quick DIY toenail trim. Like most gentlemen, he took it upon himself to cut his toenails while watching TV. During this gruesome grooming, he cut them painfully too short, uneven and with jagged edges. By being too short they began to grow inwardly and puncture the skin along the sides of the big toe developing ingrown toenails. Not being able to take the pain much longer, he allowed his lady to cut his toenails to relieve the issue. Time passed, add in some fear and painful memories, he vowed to never cut them again but leave it up to a professional. And that's how he ended up in front of me with an appointment for a pedicure!

Ingrown toenails are irregular growing toenails that grow into the skin and cut the sides of the nail bed. The most common causes are improperly cut toenails and ill-fitted shoes. The pressure applied to the sides of the feet from an inadequate shoe, with no room to move, forces the nail to grow inwardly. Plus, the foot being enclosed in a moist, dark and tight space helps to agitate a problematic situation.

Thick Toenail Treatment

Two of the most crucial culprits to many foot issues start with improperly cut toenails and ill-fitting shoes. Mentioned earlier, several feet soaks can help to soften toenails to make them easier to trim. Before trimming be sure to soak your nails for 10 minutes and dry thoroughly between toes and the nail bed. Recall dark, damp and moist environments are conducive to bacterial and fungal infections.

1. Use an emery board to file the nail going from left to right or right to left along the free edge and across the toenail to help reduce its thickness.

2. When cutting the toenails, cut just as you would when filing with an emery board. Make small cuts by sections: corner...middle...corner. This prevents jagged edged nails, chipping and splitting.

3. Smooth the nail's free edge once more with the emery board moving in one direction.

4. Use the top of the toe as your guide to determine how short the nail should be; Allowing a little free edge or white strip to be visible. Cutting the nails too short can lead to ingrown toenails and nails that puncture the skin as it begins to grow.

5. If nails are too thick and emery boards just won't do... Seek a nail professional with an electric nail drill to decrease the

nail layers and get the job done!! It's important to allow a licensed nail technician to use a drill and don't DIY. If you don't know what you're doing, drilling can lead to further nail damage and injury. Over-drilling and heat friction can be traumatic to the nail plate and lead to permanent damage.

If all else fails consider monthly pedicures! Your nail technician is equipped to cut corners (no pun intended) and see angles that you may not be flexible to view or reach. They use the proper techniques and utensils that are sterilized and effective in grooming your nails. The dedication you place on visiting your barber should be the same for nail care services. It should be a part of your grooming regiment. Like my friend and business partner Lemond Crayton-Hart says all the time "You shouldn't wear $200 J's with $3 feet".

Diabetes

The relationship between diabetes and feet is complicated. It would be careless of me if I did not dedicate a section of the book to speak on this illness. Diabetes affects the feet internally and outwardly in many serious ways. The disease damages nerves and promotes poor circulation that can lead to amputation. If not properly treated it can have damaging effects on the eyes, kidneys, nervous and immune systems, blood vessels and heart.

So...What is Diabetes? Diabetes means too much sugar in the bloodstream and not enough insulin to control its flow. With more than 29 Million Americans living with diabetes and the numbers drastically increasing, the truth is there is nothing sweet about Diabetes. Let take a moment and have a little crash course in describing the disease and how it relates to our body.

When you eat, your body turns food into sugars or glucose. This glucose is used to provide energy to the brain, body and our cells. Basically, it gives life! It's counterpart, insulin is a hormone that is made in the pancreas that helps the body store and use glucose. Its job is to be the gatekeeper and open the door of the cell allowing glucose to enter it from the bloodstream. When the body is functioning properly every cell should have an insulin hormone to escort sugar into the cell to provide it with energy. When there is not enough insulin being produced to accompany every cell or if insulin is unable to "open the door" of the cell and allow glucose in; the sugar levels rise in the bloodstream and diabetes occurs. Now there are two types of diabetes type 1 and type 2. Type I is when the pancreas doesn't produce any or enough insulin hormones for each cell to have a 1-on-1 relationship with each other. Type 1 can occur by genetics where mom and pops play a part or autoimmune when the body fights against itself. Type 2 is when the pancreas makes insulin but there is a glitch in production and insulin does not work properly. This second type is brought on by our culture and lifestyle choices pertaining to poor eating and exercise habits. In both cases, the result is high levels of sugar in the bloodstream and over time these levels become toxic. The symptoms experienced include frequent urination, excessive thirst, increased hunger, weight loss, tiredness, lack of concentration, tingling sensation or numbness felt in the hands and feet. Sounds like an infomercial to describe a new drug were you rather take your chances with the illness than deal with the side effects of using the medicine prescribed. In other words you become "HANGRY" and need a snickers.

The good news about diabetes is that it can be treated. Appropriate treatment is important in order to avoid problems with the eyes, brain, heart, kidneys, feet, and nerves. Having a healthy eating plan and doing regular exercise are keys to staying well with diabetes. In Type 1 diabetes, insulin injections are needed to control the blood sugar levels. In Type 2 diabetes, it may be tablets and/or insulin injections that may be required. In both types of diabetes, daily blood sugar checks using a meter helps to know whether the treatment plan is working or needs adjusting. Diabetes requires a team approach to keep healthy. Family working together with your doctor, diabetes educator, dietitian, and education are vital. Diabetes needs close attention but it is manageable.

I ask first-time clients if they're diabetic before beginning pedicure services. Of all the issues and problems associated with diabetes; nerve damage and poor circulation pose a serious threat to your feet. Having the information that my client is diabetic helps me to tailor my services and put their health and welfare as my highest priority. The nervous system is a highway of detailed intelligence, information, and signals that communicate directions to the body and its organs. When this system is disturbed by the effects of diabetes it's called neuropathy. Most cases of neuropathy are found in people who have diabetes. When signals can't get to the feet and lower extremities due to complications of diabetes they become numb and unresponsive.

Imagine walking and not being able to feel the ground beneath you or with every step feeling pain or a burning sensation. Constantly having to mentally calculate how to effectively maximize each step to accomplish a menial task. What would it be like if you had to turn down countless invitations because you're embarrassed cause you can't keep up with the crowd and need to lean and rest after several steps? This way of life can be scary and dangerous when dealing with the symptoms of neuropathy. Dangerous...YES! Say you step on something sharp and injure your foot. It goes unnoticed because you couldn't feel anything. Attribute poor circulation and the lack of oxygen and nutrients that don't reach the feet to begin the healing process. Over time this untreated injury can become infected and spread throughout your foot. Diabetes lowers your ability to fight infection leaving your limbs lifeless. In extreme cases amputation is needed to prevent further deterioration. In fact, 60% of patients that undergo lower-limb amputation have diabetes.

When informed that my client is diabetic I take the utmost precaution. I avoid doing anything that would puncture the skin. Doing away with any abrasive scrubs and cuticle cutting. Refrain from using any nail care equipment that is rough like pumice stones and pedicure rasp aka the foot grater directly on the thin skin. Nails are cut short but not too short to encourage ingrown, water is lukewarm and massage is given with a gentle touch. So, if you are a diabetic or know someone who is don't be afraid of getting pedicure services. Seek the recommendation of a podiatrist before undertaking any foot care treatments and solicit a knowledgeable manicurist that can provide you with a safe and quality service.

Gout

A common form of arthritis and prevalent in men; gout is an overproduction of uric acid in the blood. Uric acid is a waste product that the kidneys eliminate from the body in urine. When this waste builds up inside the body it can lead to kidney stones as well. Comparable to diabetes, when there is too much glucose in the bloodstream, gout occurs when there is too much uric acid in the blood. When uric acid levels are high it produces hard crystals that form around the joints. Most people associate gout with feet because the base of the big toe is a common joint that is affected. This build-up isn't harmful but can be painful and attack suddenly. The cause of gout goes back to lifestyle choices and lack of exercise. Your chances of getting gout are higher if your TURN UP IS REAL...meaning you enjoy too much alcohol, you're overweight and indulge in eating lots of meat and fish. Symptoms are sudden inflammation, stiffness, and swelling in your foot, ankles, knees or other joints. Attacks are sporadic and can last for a few days before the pain goes away. The prevention of the occurrence of gout and the reduction of uric acid levels begin with your diet. Limiting alcohol and sugary foods and including some gym time will help manage gout.

Foot Odor

Sweat glands in the feet produce an approximately ½ pint of perspiration daily. With 250,000 sweat glands on a pair of feet no wonder many people suffer from foot odor. The odor itself is not from the sweat; it comes from natural bacteria present in our skin that love to feast on sweat. The odor produced is the bacteria releasing gas as a byproduct. That's right: Foot odor is the results of bacteria on the feet pigging out at the sweat buffet, overeating and passing gas.

We help to encourage this flatulence of the feet by wearing closed toe shoes for hours and constantly wearing the same pair of shoes repeatedly. Also by wearing socks made of polyester and nylon material that prevent ventilation. Closed dark environments are the breeding ground for bacteria and fungus to grow and feast. So be mindful to let your shoes air out and get some fresh air on the patio. Thoroughly dry between your toes after showering or swimming. The area between your toes is a dark petri dish that can cultivate and harbor bacteria ripe for growth and infection.

Socks are a major male accessory for Men these days. Brands like Happy Socks have taken over the feet of my clients and their Instagram feeds. Even generating the hashtag #Sockwars where participants compete to see who has on the boldest, most colorfully designed, swagged-out patterned socks of the day. When choosing socks to express your style the most important characteristic is cotton. Cotton is a soft, breathable and lightweight material that's good for preventing foot odor. With today's technological advances sock are made from performance enhanced, moisture wicking fabric. These features move moisture away from the skin and spread this moisture across the fabric to enhance evaporation. Who knew socks were so intricate as if they need to be screened for

P.E.D's by the committee! So, allow the volume of your socks

to speak for you and not foot odor.

FOOT SOAKS THAT BENCH FOOT ODOR

Epsom Salt Foot Soak

An old school tried and tested foot soak with Epsom salt always wins. Not only a muscle relaxer but it kills the bacteria that feed on sweat glands that produce odor. Materials needed for this foot soak are the following:

- 8 cups of hot water and
- ½ cup of Epsom salt into the tub
- Foot tub

Soak your feet for 15-20 mins. 1-2x daily

Apple Cider Vinegar Soak

Apple cider vinegar is king when it comes to household remedies. Its acidic properties help kill bacteria, clean and disinfect foot odor and treat nail fungus. Similar to an Epsom salt soak, you'll need to soak your feet with just

- ½ cups of apple cider vinegar
- 5-8 cups of warm water
- Foot tub

Fill foot tub with all ingredients and soak for 15 minutes, twice

daily

Baking Soda and Lemon Soak

Soaking one's feet in a mixture of baking soda and the juice of

a lemon also kills bacteria, controls odor with the bonus of

softening feet. Lemon helps control excessive sweating

accompanied by a pleasant fresh scent. Ingredients needed for

this soak are as follows:

- ¼ cup of Baking soda
- 8 cups of warm water
- 1 lemon
- Foot tub/basin

Pour all ingredients into the foot tub and squeeze in the lemon

juice; Soak for 20 minutes.

Black Tea Foot Soak

Give yourself a tea party with this Black tea soak. Black tea has tannic acid that goes to war on bacteria that causes foot odor. Tannic acid is strong within the tea which kills bacteria and closes pores to help your feet sweat less. You'll need:

- 5 bags of black tea
- 4 cups of hot water
- Foot tub

Make the tea within the foot tub. Pour the hot water over the tea bags and allow them to steep for 10 minutes. Once comfortable to touch, place feet in the tub to soak for 20 minutes.

STRENGTH STRATEGIES

We spend tons of hours working out, cross fitting, kickboxing, marathon running, mountain climbing, boot camping, bodybuilding, weight training, protein shaking and putting our bodies through Insanity (pun intended). But we tend to neglect our feet which make all these activities possible. Here are a few foot exercises to help enhance your performance and relaxation tips to use when your feet are beat.

Foot Exercises

Toe Grips

Strengthens the foot muscles to improve balance.

Drop a sock on the floor and use your toes to grip and lift it off the floor. Hold for 10 seconds and repeat 5x with each foot.

Toe Extension

Strengthens and supports the muscles, which will protect the bones of the feet.

Wrap a rubber band around all five toes, double up for added tension. Expand toes and hold for 10 seconds and repeat on each foot 5x.

Calf Raises

Strengthens the feet and the calves to improve balance.

Stand near a counter, chair or wall and hold on to support your weight. With one leg lifted-up in the air. Standing on the other leg; lift yourself onto the tip of your toes and hold yourself up for 10 seconds and lower yourself down. Repeat for both calves 5x each.

Calf Stretch

Keep Achilles tendon and plantar fascia from getting tight.

You can do this one during a commercial break while sitting on the couch. Get a bathroom towel and twist it like licorice. Sit with one leg stretched out in front of you; Bend the towel in a "U" shape and place the bottom of your foot in the center while holding the ends of the towel in each hand. Gently pull the towel ends towards you until you feel a deep stretch in the arch of the foot and lower calf. Hold for 10 seconds; Release and repeat 5x for each leg.

Ankle Alphabet

Strengthen lower leg and ankle muscles. Improve ankle range of motion.

Lay down on the bed with your feet dangling over the edge.

Imagine having a piece of chalk in between your toes and

spell out the alphabet with your feet on the chalkboard. A, B,

C, D...

Foot Relaxers

Roller Massage

While sitting place a tennis ball or golf ball under your bare

feet and roll back and forth. This foot massage relieves

tension and loosens the plantar fascia.

Toe Taps

With your feet on the floor tap your toes as if you're pressing the keys on a keyboard. ASDF JKL; Embrace the toe popping it's a sign that the toes are releasing tension and build up stress.

Foot Press

With bare feet on the floor, place one foot on top of the other. Press and step on the bottom foot. Use various parts of the top foot to press different areas along the bottom foot. Take the heel of the top foot and press along the toes. Switch positions and repeat on the other foot.

Foot Twist

Sitting down (if you can) cross one leg over your thigh and wrap both hands around the foot as if you were twisting a wet dish towel. Continue this motion along the foot, twisting forward and backward. Switch feet and repeat. If it's difficult to lift your leg have someone perform the technique for you. It's a great start to a "Netflix and Chill" date night.

Toe Rotations

Sitting down (if you can) cross one leg over your thigh and hold your foot with one hand and rotate each toe in a circular motion clockwise and counter-clockwise with the other hand. Not only can you rotate each toe but also push, pull and press the toes with your hand. Repeat on the toes of the other foot.

REFLEXOLOGY

*"Most people have no idea how good their body
is designed to feel" -Kevin Trudeau*

Relatively new to western civilization and popular culture; Reflexology is the practice of applying pressure to specific points and areas on the feet, hands, and face to relieve tension and restore balance. It's believed that these areas and reflex points are outwardly located on the body to "reflect and mirror" the actual internal organs and body systems. By applying pressure to these areas with a specific thumb and finger technique, the recipient will enjoy positive effects on the organs and their overall health. A traditional wisdom that has been around for about 5000 years documented in the histories of China and Egypt; Reflexology is more than a foot massage it's an alternative medicine that can rejuvenate energy, relieve stress and tension, release chemicals such as endorphins to unblock negativity and bring about positive results for your overall health.

I was introduced to Reflexology in search of adding more services for my clients to enjoy. Through a google search on foot care, I came across the practice, did my research and believed it was a way to add value to my business. I was so intrigued I found a local practitioner in my city who was quite knowledgeable and confident about her craft. I chose the blue pill and immediately signed up for the 1200 hours course...never to look back.

In my short experience with Reflexology, I'll describe it as a way to hit the reset button and encourage the body to find balance. I have conducted sessions with clients and the results have been undeniable. I've witnessed congestion, sinus pressure and migraine tension dissipate. After having rotator cuff surgery, Reflexology helped accelerate the healing process of a client and was verified by their doctor. Menstrual cycles have normalized, bowels unblocked and the list goes on! Even though the scientific community does not recognize Reflexology as an effective treatment for any medical condition I am a believer that it's real and I have proof!!

I have found that before an ailment will manifest itself outwardly it first will be revealed on the feet. Our feet are forever changing, just as we grow mentally, physically, spiritually and emotionally our "soles" are also evolving as well.

The benefits of Reflexology are endless and I wish more people would take advantage of this holistic bodywork especially Men. Like most self-care practices a lot of men don't think pampering is masculine. However, there are many reasons why men should consider carving out some "Me Time" and take the advice of Aaron Rodgers the QB of the Green Bay Packers "R-E-L-A-X...Relax". It's a vital part of your total wellness.

"Caring for myself is not self-indulgence, it is self-preservation and that is an act of political warfare." – Audre Lorde

One last point that might peak your interest to learn more about the therapy...SEX!!! Reflexology has all the benefits of sex and so much more. Like sex, Reflexology brings about great joy and a fresh new perspective on life:

- It helps to keep your immune system humming

- boost your libido to enjoy more lively sex

- lowers blood pressure

- burns calories

- lowers your risk of heart attack

- lessens pain by activating endorphins

- lessens your chance of getting prostate cancer

- enhances your sleep

- eases stress and anxiety

Reflexology has all these advantages and MUCH MORE!

ALPHAMALE AFFIRMATIONS:
YOUR STEPS ARE ORDERED

"I AM two of the most powerful words. For what you put after them shapes your reality" -Author Unknown

I never knew that I would be an Entrepreneur, Small Business Owner or New York Times Bestseller (speaking that last one into existence). The plan I set for myself was to graduate from college, get a GOOD job and live happily ever after. Hopeful that marriage, kids, and traveling would be included. Never could I imagine I would experience 2 lay-offs and a termination which were all designed in hindsight to lead me to my true purpose. Regardless of all that has transpired I always maintained my faith, a positive attitude, and a GOOD word.

"Words Cast Spells, that's Why it's Called Spelling Words"

There is power in every word that you speak. When we speak we activate life or death. Each one of us has the spirit of God residing within us and are made in HIS image! When HE speaks things happen...worlds were framed, life was created, miracles manifested! This same principle is applicable to our lives whether you believe it or not. We have been given the same authority and dominion to ask and speak what we want and to believe that we will receive. It's a universal law that works every time!

When I decided to transition from confining corporate cubicles to full-time entrepreneurship I was scared as hell. Nothing can really prepare you for stepping out on faith into unknown and risky territory. I took no business classes, had no examples of entrepreneurial role models...just a few books, Google, and a passion. During this season I gained great inspiration from sermons and scriptures. One particular sermon spoke on the passage of Luke 7:36-50. At that time, I was at a crossroad and needed direction, clarity, and confirmation. Fear caused me to doubt and question if I was walking in my purpose. The Universe always has a way of giving you the answers you seek when you ask. This parable got my full attention when I heard that this woman gave Jesus a pedicure because she was so grateful and humbled by the love and forgiveness he had shown her. In honor of him, she washed his feet with her tears and dried them with her hair. This scripture affirmed the foundation for my business model and how I wanted to treat every client I encountered...with honor, respect and love. This passage gave me my WHY...when passion isn't enough and I want to give up. I always find grace in Luke 7:37-50.

I AM THE WOMAN WITH THE ALABASTER BOX.

I spend an astronomical amount of time with feet: cutting, clipping, massaging and researching. I'm very attentive to the look, texture, and character of a person's feet. My fixation with all things feet began to consume me with how often within our daily lives we reference the foot and its many capabilities:

A runaway bride – **She had cold FEET**

Talking too much and offend someone – **He put his FOOT in his mouth**

Fall in Love -**Head over HEELS; Swept me off me FEET**

Getting Ready to Compete – **Go TOE to TOE**

Procrastinating – **Dragging your FEET**

Starting Something That's Likely to Fail – **Get off on the wrong FOOT**

Horrible Dancer – **Dancing with two left FEET**

Exercising Patience – **One STEP at a time**

To Be Independent – **Stand on your own two FEET**

Causing Yourself Problems – **Shoot yourself in the FOOT**

Be Alert and Ready – **On your TOES**

Perspective – **Shoe is on the other FOOT**

Come Back from a Setback – **Get back on your FEET**

To Resign or Retire – **STEP aside**

Make a Good Impression – **Put your best FOOT forward**

Try Something New- **Get your FEET wet**

Hurry Up – **STEP on it**

Adventurous Risk Taker- **Take a WALK on the wild side;**

It doesn't stop there!!! The symbolism of "feet", "walk" and "steps" are also powerfully present in scripture. It has greatly impacted spirituality and has helped to make the Bible and its principles practical.

After digging into the scriptures my WHY became personal and greater than me. It's more than manicures and pedicures... it's my service. And I have an attitude of gratitude.

I've been chosen to wash the feet of Kings and serve the

Children of GOD aka "the Kids".

> *A man's gift makes room for him and brings*
> *him before great men. -Proverbs 18:16*

I began to understand how valuable feet are and the

power they possess. With each pedicure, I'm transferring

energy through touch, so it's vital that I feast on positivity and

speak, think and walk in the light.

> *"Service to others is the rent you pay for your room*
> *here on earth"* -Muhammad Ali

During my time with each client, I take advantage of

this appointed time to speak life over each set of feet that are

before me! I like to hashtag these words on social media as

#AlphaMaleAffirmations. Affirmations can change your life!!!

These positive statements communicate with Yourself and the Spirit, GOD, Atmosphere, Universe... (whomever you believe) what you desire to see take place in your life. What you THINK about is what you'll SPEAK about and that will soon encourage you into ACTION! You'll begin to move in that direction! The energy you put forth will be met by a UNANIMOUS FORCE of FAVOR to help you accomplish every word, thought and action that was spoken. God said, "Let there be light...and there was light". This super natural power belongs to you; passed down to The Kids from your Father!!

A - B - R - A - C - A - D - A - B - R - A

Abracadabra in Hebrew means "It came to pass as it was spoken"

Recognize the truth that life and death are in the power of YOUR tongue...CHOOSE LIFE! Get in the habit of speaking to your future in the present. Be patient... it's a process but well worth the wait. You'll be amazed at the manifestation of your spoken words becoming a reality.

"Speak Now or Forever Hold Your Peace"

I get asked all the time "How did you come up with the business name?" Like most people I asked Google. "Okay Google...What are synonyms for masculinity?" Of all the suggested words "ALPHAMALE" captured the essence of the brand I wanted to create. The definitions, articles, images, videos and current affairs assured my decision. ALPHA is the beginning, likewise the concept and vision for nail care services for men was the first of its kind. As I began to study the word; the letters "A" and "M" caught my attention. "I AM" are the two most powerful words on Earth!!

What do you think about Yourself? I stated earlier "How you describe your feet is a direct reflection of the life you live." Positive outcomes are linked to positive thinking. The same is true for negative thoughts. Your experiences will resemble your thoughts, words and actions.

To prove a point, let's talk about the 2018 Super Bowl Champions. The entire 2017 NFL season headlined and captioned the Philadelphia Eagles as the underdog. With the odds and opinions stacked against them, their locker room interviews and press conferences remained consistent "Faith and Football". The team and staff chose to focus their thoughts and abilities on winning and being on the same frequency for 17 weeks. To everyone's surprise the underdogs made it to Super Bowl LII. The opponents...the iconic, legendary, 5x Super Bowl champions The New England Patriots. The game was a classic David and Goliath match-up. Although I was impartial to the outcome I secretly wished for all the Meek Mill's and Kevin Hart's of the world that the Eagles would claim victory. The game was a thrilling "nail-biter" with a series of favorable calls for the Eagles. As the fans sang in unison "Fly, Eagles Fly" the score was 41 -33 and the Philadelphia Eagles won their first Super Bowl.

It goes to show your dreams can come true with a positive mindset in conjunction with encouraging self-talk and a team of like-minded individuals. "I AM" statements help you to reprogram your thoughts to break patterns of doubt and fear. Repetition of these short phrases will begin to marinate into your subconscious and "abracadabra" the results will be as you desire. You can change your reality with positive affirmations. Learning to control your thoughts and words takes discipline. But mastering this skill will improve your world tremendously.

When practicing affirmations you must be clear about your intentions. Avoid toxic words that could sabotage the process like can't, don't, won't or not. Repeat, repeat, repeat both verbally and in writing. The more you visualize and hear yourself speaking life the mind will start to believe it and you will achieve it. Below are a few "AlphaMale" affirmations to help you begin the practice of positive self -talk.

AlphaMale Affirmations

I AM Powerful

I AM Confident

I AM Blessed

I AM Wealthy

I AM Healthy

I AM a Leader

I AM Loved

I AM Grateful

I AM Patient

I AM at Peace with Myself

I AM Alphamale

RECIPES AND REMEDIES: ESSENTIAL OILS 101

*"The greatest medicine of all is to teach people
how not to need it" - Hippocrates*

Okay... I'm sure the subject of essential oils is not the topic of discussion in the locker room or tailgate. Usually, women are more interested in essential oils and their medicinal and cleansing properties. But allow me to convince you that essential oils add great value to the user.

The concentrated essences of various flowers, fruits, herbs, and plants have been used across many cultures around the world for centuries. Modern scientific research has proven that essential oils are potent and powerful with benefits far beyond their sweet fragrance. Evidence and recorded history show that Egyptians were renowned for their knowledge of cosmetology, ointments and aromatic oils. Priest, Kings, and Pharaohs (All Men of Course) during this period created various blends to treat illness, to meditate and for perfumes. It was considered a privilege to be allowed to use these oils and regarded necessary to be one with God. Warriors brought essential oils to battle, to treat infection and to use during massages before war to help them relax and focus. Essential oils have played an important role in society for both genders. They boast a plethora of benefits to our mental, physical and spiritual being. Essential oils can be a crucial part of your arsenal to help you heal holistically without damaging side effects and toxins.

Steering away from commercial products made with fillers and synthetic chemicals that have been linked to various cancers; I've compiled a list of recipes and remedies that are convenient, DIY with a masculine appeal. Enjoy!!

Men usually tend to gravitate towards earthy, spicy and woody flavors. Some recommended oils that are considered quintessential fragrances for men are:

Patchouli	**Sandalwood**	**Oakmoss**
Bay Rum	**Lavender**	**Ginger**
Black Pepper	**Vanilla**	**Jasmine**
	Cypress	

Patchouli
Description: rich, earthy, woody aroma

Uses: acne, athlete's foot, chapped skin, dermatitis, eczema, fatigue, frigidity, hair care, insect repellant, mature skin, oily skin, stress.

Sandalwood
Description: rich, sweet, fragrant yet delicate, woody, floral.

Uses: acne, depression, skin Infections, fungal and bacterial Infections, stress, aphrodisiac

Oakmoss
Description: rich, earthy, woody

Uses: adds an earthy aroma to fragrances

Bay Rum
Description: medicinal, fruity, spicy, herbaceous aroma.

Uses: cold and flu, hair care, poor circulation, sprains, strains.

Cypress
Description: Fresh, herbaceous, slightly woody, evergreen aroma.

Uses: Excessive perspiration, hemorrhoids, oily skin, concentration, astringent

Ginger
Description: Warm, spicy, earthy, woody.

Uses: Aching muscles, arthritis, nausea, poor circulation, sprains, digestive disorder

Black Pepper
Description: Crisp, fresh, woody, peppercorn aromas

Uses: Colds, Aches and Pain, Influenza, alertness, and stamina, muscle cramps

Vetiver
Description: Woody, smoky, earthy, herbaceous and spicy

Uses: Nervousness, muscular relaxant, cuts, acne, depression, Insomnia, Antiseptic

Other Masculine Essential Oils
(earthy, spicy, sporty, woody)

Ambrette Seed, Angelica Root, Amyris, Anise

Balsam (Peru), Basil, Bay, Bay Laurel, Beeswax, Benzoin, Bergamot, Blue Cypress

Cajeput, Cananga, Caraway Seed, Cardamom, Carrot Seed, Cedarwood (Atlas), Cedarwood (Virginian), Cinnamon, Clary Sage, Coriander, Cypress, Cypress (Blue)

Davana

Fennel, Fir Needle, Frankincense

Ginger, Grapefruit, Gurjum Balsam

Helichrysum, Holy Basil, Hyssop

Immortelle

Juniper Berry

Kanuka

Lime

Mandarin, Manuka, Marjoram, May Chang, Melissa, Mullein, Myrrh, Myrtle, Myrtle (Lemon)

Neroli, Nutmeg

Oakmoss, Orange (Bitter), Orange (Sweet), Oregano

Palo Santo, Parsley, Patchouli, Pepper (Black), Petitgrain, Pine (Scotch)

Sage (Spanish), Sandalwood, Spruce, Star Anise

Tagetes, Tangerine, Thyme, Tobacco

Vanilla, Vetiver

Citrus oils are also popular amongst
blends preferred by men:

Orange   **Tangerine**   **Lemon**

                        Lime   **Grapefruit**

Orange (Sweet/Bitter)
Description: Citrusy, sweet,

Uses: Depression, Colds, constipation, muscular
                 spasm, antiseptic

Lime
Description: Fresh, citrusy, sweet, slightly tart.

Uses: Fevers, acne, asthmas, sore throat,
                 headaches, depression, flu, antiseptic,
                 antiviral

Grapefruit
Description: Citrusy. Tangy and sweet

Uses: Obesity, Kidney and Liver problems,
                 Migraines, Depression

Top 16 Essential Oils

Bergamot
Eucalyptus
Grapefruit
Lemon
Lime
Peppermint
Rosemary
Tangerine

Cinnamon Leaf
Frankincense
Lavender
Lemongrass
Patchouli
Pine Needle
Sweet Orange
Tea Tree

Essential oils in a pure state can be too harsh for direct skin contact. You'll need to dilute these concentrated oils and mix with a base oil or more commonly known as carrier oils. Carrier oils are so named because they "Carry" the oils on the skin. Examples of good carrier oil is a product that can be massaged into the skin and/or hair. A good carrier oil needs to be rich in protein and good for all skin types:

Popular Carrier Oils
Almond Oil
Grapeseed Oil
Jojoba Oil
Carrot Oil
Sesame Oil
Olive Oil
Sunflower Oil

Note: For every 5 drops of essential oil add 1 teaspoon of

carrier oil

Foot Care Recipes Using Essential Oils
(Blend all Recipes with Your Choice of Carrier Oil)

Foot Rejuvenator Blend (use for foot massage)
Lavender
Peppermint
Rosemary

Bunions, Blisters, Corns & Calluses
Tagetes
Jojoba Oil
Carrot Oil

Black Toe Nail

Hyssop
Foot Odor Powder
Tea Tree
Sage
Baking Powder

Ingrown Toe Nail
Lavender
Tea Tree

Diabetes
Cinnamon
Coriander
Clove
Myrrh
Cypress
Lavender

Cuticle Softener
Jojoba Oil
Carrot Oil
Eucalyptus
Peppermint

Nail Infections
Tea Tree
Eucalyptus
Lavender
Oregano

Achilles Tendinitis
Cypress
Rosemary
Frankincense
Lavender
Ginger
Eucalyptus
Peppermint

Nail Strengthener

Lemon
Lavender
Eucalyptus
Peppermint
Carrot
Rosemary
Cypress
Patchouli
Tagetes
Grapefruit

Stress Fractures

Lavender
Thyme
Ginger
Geranium

SHOE GAME GUIDELINES

"It's Great to be Known for Your Shoes,
But it's Better to be Known for your Sole."
– Kenneth Cole

It's said you can tell a lot about a man by his shoes!

Mentioned earlier, shoes are a major factor in foot ailments

and responsible for many issues that later manifest due to

improper fit. Footwear impacts your posture, how you walk

and how you represent yourself. So how is your shoe game? Do

you rock hard bottoms to the 9 to 5 or are you a "sneaker-

head" with a pair of retro Air Jordan balling at the gym? Do you

switch it up with comfortable crocs on a lazy Sunday afternoon

or does your workwear include a pair of heavy-duty steel toes

boots? Whatever the occupation, event or activity it's vital that

your shoes are always on point; with the primary focus on fit and comfort rather than just style. Below are a few tips to keep in mind on your next shoe shopping trip:

The size of your feet changes as you grow older so always have your feet measured before buying shoes. The best time to shop for shoes is afternoon/evening that's when your feet are at their largest. Most of us have one foot that is larger than the other. Fit and purchase shoes according to the larger foot.

Before purchasing shoes always base your decision on fit and comfort. It's not enough to just assume it's your right size because its marked on the box, shoe tag or available online. Save time by trying shoes on. Different brands and styles have different cuts. Your size 12 may fit cozy in an Aldo but be too roomy in a Cole Haan; Adidas may fit like a glove but Puma might be sliding off the heel.

During the fitting process make sure there is enough space to fit your longest toe while standing up. Leaving 3/8 to ½ inch space from the tip of the toe to the end of the shoe.

Never leave the store with the expectation that the shoe will stretch to fit. There will be a little expansion overtime but comfort is key before you purchase. Leather will expand and widen with multiple wears but only a little bit. However, shoes will not lengthen.

Make sure the ball of your foot agrees with the widest part of the shoe as the ball is the widest part of your foot.

Bring with you the type of socks you would normally wear with a particular style of shoe when shopping. In other words, avoid wearing dress socks trying on sneakers.

Take note of how your heels sit in the shoe. If it slips out while testing the shoe chances are they will continue to do so. The soles will become more flexible with wear and will slightly alleviate this problem. The source of this issue is that many shoes have too wide of a heel, to begin with.

Walk around the store in both the left and right shoe before buying and once more at home a few hours on a surface that will not scuff the soles. This should give you a better feel and a better chance to be able to return them if they don't work out.

Now let's focus on Style and Fashion:

When choosing which pair of shoes to wear out, try to pick a pair that matches or is darker than your pants.

Try to match your shoe color with the color of your belt.

Jeans allow versatility when it comes to shoes. Any color and style of shoe will not conflict with a pair of jeans.

Socks should be a bridge between your pants and shoes.

There are an incredible amount of colors and patterns of socks as well as colored shoestrings that can add character to your #OOTD (outfit of the day). Have fun expressing your individuality and maintain consistency when coordinating.

Have multiple pairs of black shoes...black tend to go with everything!

Please NO SOCK WITH SANDALS

Shoes All Men Must Have:

- Formal Dress Shoe: Black/Navy/ Brown- Good to have when attending your Frat Brothers Wedding and formal occasions

- Athletic Cross-trainer shoe for working out

- Sandals for warmer weather and vacation

- Comfortable Casual Shoe for the office use or the everyday go-to shoe like a Loafer.

- Dressy Casual Shoe when you need to step it up for date night but don't want to seem over the top and formal

- Lifestyle Shoe that's sporty to catch a game with the fellas or little league practice with the kids.

- A good pair of boots.

Learn how to shine your shoes or find a professional shoe shiner. We'll revisit this point later. Replace your workout shoes at least every 6 months and have a couple pairs to switch into during this time frame. This helps to prevent injuries and gives your shoes time to air out. This method also discourages fungus and bacteria growth that could lead to infection as well as increases the shelf life of your shoes.

THE ART OF SHOE SHINING

"If both of your shoes are shined, then your
best foot will always be forward"
- Maryrose Wood

Every Man should know how to shine his shoes and you don't need a military background to learn. It's a good skill to acquire and speaks volumes to the type of man you are and the standards you possess. Like my business partner and friend LeMond always says, "Treat yourself like a King and everyone else will do the same!" Shining your shoes is like polishing the diamonds on your crown. Not only does it make them look more presentable when putting your best foot forward; it cleans, conditions and extends the life of your favorite pair of shoes.

All the things you'll need to properly shine your shoes can be found in a shoe shine kit. If this isn't readily available, four essential items you need to get started are a tin of shoe polish, a horsehair shoe brush, two soft and clean cloths (one to apply polish and another to buff); and a toothbrush on deck for the hard to reach spots.

Step 1: Gather Your Supplies

Tins of shoe polish are available in a variety of colors. Choose the polish that closely resembles your shoe leather. Shoe polish comes in both wax and cream and there are mixed reviews about wax vs cream polish. But of course, it all comes down to preference.

Wax vs Cream Polish

Wax based polish will produce a superior shine and has the added value of waterproofing the shoe. A liability to using wax is that it clogs the pores of the leather. Be mindful that leather should be treated like skin because it is a skin! Like skin, it needs to breathe, be cleansed and moisturized. When your skin is clogged with oil and dirt it produces acne. Similar, when leather absorbs grit and grime it cracks, becomes abrasive and breaks down. When using too much wax it disables the ability for leather to breathe. You wouldn't walk around with dry cracked skin on your hands, lips, and elbows...so why would you walk around with dry visibly cracked and creased shoes? On the other hand, shoe cream is a leather conditioner and penetrates deeper into the leather. A drawback of cream polish is that it produces a moderate shine in comparison to wax based polish. If possible use both by alternating between polishes to get the best of both worlds.

As stated earlier you'll need two soft cloths, one to apply polish and one to buff. This material can come from an old white tee or a chamois just make sure it's clean. Shoe polish can be extremely difficult to remove so to avoid smearing polish on the floor or furniture, lay an old newspaper or an old towel on your work surface. Get comfortable and put on your favorite playlist! Shoe shining can take some time and if you're like me you pay close attention to details.

Step 2: Clean and Condition the Shoes

Clean the dust and dirt off your shoes with the horsehair brush; For hard, stuck on dirt use a damp rag. It's important to remove all dirt before polishing because leftover or overlooked particles can scratch the leather surface during the polishing phase. Saddle soap is recommended to clean, condition and protect the leather. Just like any soap, dampen a cloth and mix into the soap tin to produce a lather and apply to the shoes.

After cleaning the shoes let them dry completely before moving to the next step.

Step 3: Apply Shoe Polish

Now it's time to polish. Get started by placing a little water in the lid of the tin can of polish to dampen your cloth. Wrap a portion of your clean cloth or t-shirt around the forefingers of the hand that will be applying polish. For some sturdiness and to have better control, place the other hand inside of the shoe. Apply polish evenly to the surface of the shoe.

Most shoe shine kits supply a circular shoe polish sponge that is effective too. Just make sure you have different sponges for each tin color. Use circular motions to work the polish into every part of the shoe. Remove shoestrings if applicable in order to reach the "tongue" of the shoe. Bring out the toothbrush for hard to reach areas and seams. Allow 15 mins for polish to dry, as a bonus place them in the sun. The sun adds value by melting the polish and helping it to evenly distribute on the shoe for a better shine. And with leather being a type of "skin" vitamin D is a benefit for the shoes and an opportunity to air them out while outside. For a personal touch just use your fingertips to apply the polish in a circular motion. This method also helps warm the wax to soften it for better application.

Step 4: Remove Excess Polish

Once the polish is dry, you can begin to remove the excess using the horsehair brush. Horsehair bristles are commonly used because they are soft and will not damage or scratch the leather surface. It's important, if possible, to use a different brush for each colored polish as it helps to prevent cross-contamination from color to color. Make sure the brush is clean from its previous duty of removing visible dust and dirt from the shoes. Brush the entire shoe vigorously using short even strokes for better coverage. The friction created during this step will help any remaining polish to "sink" into the leather grain and give you an even shine. Use the toothbrush to remove excess from the tiny cracks and crevices or use a clean q-tip! Repeat steps 4 & 5 on the heel and toe areas as these locations see a lot of creasing.

Step 5: Buff the Shoes with a Cloth

Take the other cloth or chamois cloth, buff the shoe until you achieve the high shine you like. Use a brisk side to side motion to buff the top and a "U" shape motion to shine the heel and the sides of the shoes. Want that Rhianna "shine bright like a diamond" result? A military tip is to buff with a nylon stocking to achieve that superior shine. During this part, it may be easier to put the shoe on for some stability and support it by stepping onto a shoe caddy. Give extra attention to the toe area since this portion gets high visibility. A "spit -shine" can be duplicated with a few splashes of water and continue buffing.

Step 6: Repeat all the above steps on the other shoe.

Once you get into your shoe shining groove you'll adjust and tweak these steps to fit your needs. This is just a simple beginner's method to get you started.

As a side note to all the shoe enthusiast: invest in a few wooden shoe trees! High-quality shoe trees are made of wood. Used to extend the life of the shoe, shoe trees preserve its shape and stop it from developing creases. Although many kinds of wood are used to make shoe trees, cedar is the most popular. It has the added value of being able to absorb sweat that could damage the interior of the shoe and lead to a rotting lining. Think about your cigar humidor! Most likely it is made of cedar wood for its ability to protect the cigars, retain their character and freshness, and regulate the atmosphere. Cedar works the same towards your shoes as well as tackles foot odor. And with what you've learned about essential oils, a perfect gift could be a set of shoe trees treated with your very own custom essential oil blends using oils that boast antiviral and antibacterial properties. Also, find a nearby shoe repair shop with a good Cobbler; he will be able to preserve your shoes by resoling them and add taps to ensure longevity.

#MANICURESMATTER

Title: Weak Handshake
Artist: Captee

Weak handshake
your fake
part snake
your eyes are not in-line with mine
hate
where is the love?
I extended to bring in
oppose to a shove
a friend I'm thinking
but what I know from above
is how to determine
damn near deferring
the "her" in "him"
because in
3 to 5 seconds I'm dissecting your characteristics
from grip to stance
even that quick to the left glance
the position of your right hand
the expand of your pupils
let's me know that you're not truthful
the damned in a dam
over ran by the ills of man
damn
am I asking for too much?
but for brothers to keep it all the way at a 100
when they touch
this man's hands

Because this man's hands are used to provide
and chastise
test my manhood
and I'll crinkle and crumble a couple of
knuckles off the lambs hove
Handshakes are sometimes signed
contracts in the absents of ink
your projected abstract is absent
to the brawn with brains that thinks
I think
matter fact I know
that you gotta come correct
or your hidden agenda will show
the Baboons foe expose with a gaussian glow
neon green is the hue
blue in the cold
if your eyes are the windows to your soul
for sure
then your handshake is the welcome mat
to its door

I would be remiss if I did not mention manicures. It is a must-have accessory to any grooming regiment. Manicures add value to your overall presentation. It makes no sense rockin' a rolly, rolly, rolly with a dab of ranch...and some ice on your wrist with some jacked-up hands!!! Or sporting a Cartier with claws as fingernails. The two just don't match and you took an "L" on the investment.

May I pose a question: How many times did you shake someone's hand or gave someone dap today? Think about all the people you've had physical contact with and had to introduce yourself with a handshake or a hug. Handshakes are a crucial aspect in how we brand ourselves to the world. They carry a lot of weight in forming how others view you for the first time. Handshakes are a powerful tool to communicate confidence, trust, and self-worth in a matter of moments.

*   *   *

I had the privilege to be a chosen vendor for the National League of Cities (NLC for short). According to their IG account, NLC is an organization that "represents cities of all sizes, from rural communities and growing suburbs to the largest cities". Annually they host conferences in major cities across the country and their 2017 City Summit was hosted by the "Queen City" at the Convention Center.

Hundreds of city officials, mayors and councilmen descended upon my city. They had three days to meet and greet, talk about the "mess" they have going on in their respective cities, get some money and hopefully find a solution to clean up the "Shit in the City"!!

The House of LeMond and myself had a personal invitation from the former President of the NLC Committee Board to be in attendance. The stipulations were to pay $99 to represent Charlotte's small business community in what they called the Market Square. Us and 19 other local businesses for the duration of the summit would provide a retail experience for the visitors. According to the rules, we were asked to bring up to 100 pounds of goods and materials that we wished to

showcase and sell. The stats stated that the city officials in

attendance would represent 19,000 cities, towns and villages

encompassing 49 states. And did I mention Magic Johnson was

going to be the keynote speaker!!!

Our daily mantra at The House of LeMond is "Say Less

and Think Vast"!!! What's the odds that one of these city

council (wo)men or mayors at this summit could be the next

President of the USA? If #45 (his name will go unmentioned)

can be POTUS surely one of these individuals has what it

takes!!!!

I had an amazing opportunity to highlight the business:

"rub shoulders" or more so massage the hands of city leaders

from all over the country. Take some pictures for the 'gram,

MAKE SOME MONEY and possibly see Magic Johnson? HELL YEAH!!! We RSVP'ed immediately!

As a Market Square vendor, my team created the quintessential gentlemen's pop-up shop. Men are never really considered at these events. Nothing in the "thanks for coming" recycle-able swag bag includes a gift for guys. So that's what we brought—100lbs of clothing, men's specialty goods, leather handmade bags, oils, dope ass socks and shoe accessories, custom garments, blazers, and bowties…we had it ALL!! And for the extra point, shoeshines and manicure services were available on-site. Before we could finish setting up a line had formed.

Lunch was like timeouts between mastermind meetings, workshops and panel discussions. Guests gathered around waiting for their turn to get buffed and shined. During these mini manicure moments, I sparked up a conversation with a skeptic on the topic of manicures for men. I shared with him the same question I posed to you earlier: How many times have you shaken hands today? While he contemplated the answer, my touch put a spell on him like Nina Simone! He mumbled inaudible sounds of pleasure as I stretched, bent and pulled his fingers. His hands "popped locked and dropped" as I kneaded every pressure point. Putting the finishing touches on his manicure; he opened his eyes and examined my work. Astonished by the instant gratification and the drastic before and after, this skeptic turned into a believer. Before he departed he dropped a chunky tip in my repurposed cigar box. As he gathered his things I said "The YES you've been waiting for might be on the other side of that manicure. #ManicuresMatter"! With a nod of the head in agreement, he walked away rubbing his hands like Birdman. I watched him leave and thought "... 'cause you're mine" another satisfied customer! Again, I say- "on the other side of your manicure could be the opportunity you've been waiting and praying for". Think VAST you've got the whole world in your hands!!!

"Whose world is this? The world is yours" -Nas

Just recently I had a speaking engagement with Wake Forest's MBA program on the topic of Branding. During my 30 minutes set I specified that you should cover all five senses: taste, sight, smell, sound, and touch when it comes to communicating who you are. Branding is just finding a way to communicate who you are so others clearly understand. When it comes to the sense of touch, I use this teachable moment to plug the manicures matter movement as I shake the hands of those closest to the front. I'll share with you what I told the students: You have five senses and seven seconds to grab the audience's attention!! What the F*ck can you do in 7 seconds?

The "Seven Second Rule" came from a TV executive my team and I had the pleasure of speaking with while filming a pilot episode in Atlanta. The gentleman discussed with us facts and tactics used in the world of tv production. He told us that the average person skips channels at the rate of seven seconds. Even though I cut the cable years ago I could relate to playlist surfing on my iPhone until I heard the right song. I would skip so much on Pandora I just went ahead and bought a monthly subscription to take advantage of unlimited skips and no commercials.

Are you skippable or memorable? When you greet opportunity are your hands dry, cracked and callused with a side dish of hangnails? Do your fingertips look like you've been gnawing and feasting on them like finger food? Or do you announce yourself with confidence, showcasing hands that could seal million-dollar deals! Shaking hands allows you to enter someone's personal space and vice versa. The invitation into your space should be personable; not cold and awkward with stuff all over the place as you scramble to tidy up.

Plain and simple a manicure means to care for your hands. The DIY method is as follows:

1.   Clipping and cutting nails no shorter than your fingernails.

2.   Shape and file the nails to frame your fingers.

3.   File in one direction from left to right and not back and forth.

4.   Clean any dirt or debris that has collected under the nail.

5.   Wash, dry and moisturize.

We use our hands daily and they are visible in all that we do. You may not realize it but you probably "talk" with your hands. A study conducted by researchers "Science of People" analyzed thousands of hours of TED talks. They discovered the most viral Talkers spoke with their hands. The most popular Ted Talkers used an average of 465 hand gestures during the 18-minute talk. Researchers have found that those who "talk" with their hands are viewed as charismatic, agreeable and energetic.

Other facts that came from the study:

- Hand gestures make people listen and pay attention to you. Using your hands helps the listener be more engaged with the sounds of your words and the visual movement of your hands helps to stimulate other senses that encourage focus.

- Gesturing helps you to access stored memories and refresh your thoughts so you speak fluidity and effectively.

- Gestures increase the value of your message by 60%

If I still haven't persuaded you, allow me to shoot my shot one last time. The root word in manicure is MAN!!! C'mon Man, what else do I need to say to convince you to make the right investment. Invest in Yourself and be the MAN in manicures!!! #ManicuresMatter

ALPHAMALE AFTERWORDS:
THE CROWNING MOMENT

When your treat yourself like a King everyone and everything will follow your lead!

"Raw Footage: A Gentlemen's Guide to Proper Foot Care" is just my way of helping you to adjust your crown. But it's up to you to polish, protect and claim your position on the throne. Embrace the power to create your own gold standard of Masculinity. Understanding that "Health is Wealth" and your wellbeing should not be compromised due to the opinions of others. You deserve to live abundantly in every aspect of your life.

I hope the information shared has planted a seed within you to place more emphasis on how you treat yourself; especially your feet. Self-care can be overwhelming at the beginning but start with what feels good to you. The path will manifest once you decide to shift your focus to what you really want. Soon you'll be asking yourself what took so long for you to arrive to this place of solace. Remember to walk by faith and present your best foot forward knowing all your steps are ordered!

Peace!

Bibliography

Bible verses, retrieved from The Holy Bible (NKJV)

Chapter: AlphaMale Affirmations: Your Steps Are Ordered

Worwood, Valerie Ann. The Complete Book of Essential Oils & Aromatherapy

Chapter: Foot Soaks that Bench Foot Odor

Chapter: Recipes and Remedies: Essential Oils 101

https://www.scienceofpeople.com/hand-gestures/

Chapter: #ManicuresMatter

Press Conference With Sheena Pickett

Sheena C. Pickett is a mathematician, entrepreneur, small business owner, and self-published author. When she's not playing with feet, you can find her with a good book moderating cool, co-ed conversations as the host of *Satire Sunday: A Co-ed Book Club*. She resides in Charlotte, North Carolina supporting local community organizations such as The Men's Shelter of Charlotte and Samaritans Feet.

Visit AlphaMale Nail Care Services website:

www.alphamalenailcare.com

www.ingramcontent.com/pod-product-compliance
Lightning Source LLC
Chambersburg PA
CBHW031400250726
48656CB00002B/508